Healthy Slow Cooker Cookbook

Easy Slow Cooker Recipes for Keep Health and Lose Weight

By Robin Ellgen

Sommario

Introduction

We understand you are constantly searching for much easier methods to prepare your dishes. We additionally know you are possibly sick and tired of investing lengthy hours in the kitchen cooking with numerous pans and pots. Well, now your search mores than! We located the best kitchen area tool you can make use of from now on! We are discussing the Slow stove! These remarkable pots allow you to cook a few of the very best dishes ever before with minimum initiative Sluggish stoves prepare your meals simpler and also a lot much healthier! You do not require to be a professional in the kitchen to prepare a few of the most delicious, flavored, textured and abundant meals! All you need is your Slow cooker and the appropriate active ingredients! This wonderful recipe book you are about to discover will certainly educate you how to prepare the best slow-moving cooked dishes. It will reveal you that you can make some impressive breakfasts, lunch meals, side dishes, poultry, meat as well as fish meals. Finally yet notably, this recipe book gives you some basic and also wonderful treats.

Chili Eggs Mix

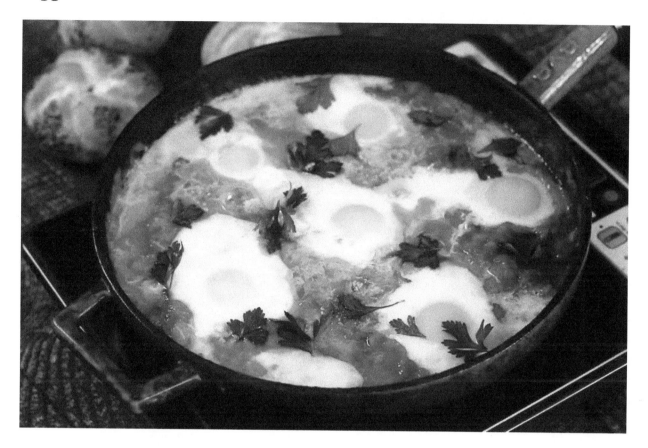

Preparation time: 10 minutes
Cooking time: 3 hours
Servings: 2

Ingredients:
- Cooking spray
- 3 spring onions, chopped
- 2 tablespoons sun dried tomatoes, chopped
- 1 ounce canned and roasted green chili pepper, chopped
- ½ teaspoon rosemary, dried
- Salt and black pepper to the taste
- 3 ounces cheddar cheese, shredded
- 4 eggs, whisked
- ¼ cup heavy cream
- 1 tablespoon chives, chopped

Directions:
1. Grease your slow cooker with cooking spray and mix the eggs with the chili peppers and the other ingredients except the cheese.

2. Toss everything into the pot, sprinkle the cheese on top, put the lid on and cook on High for 3 hours.
3. Divide between plates and serve.

Nutrition: calories 224, fat 4, fiber 7, carbs 18, protein 11

Chocolate Breakfast Bread

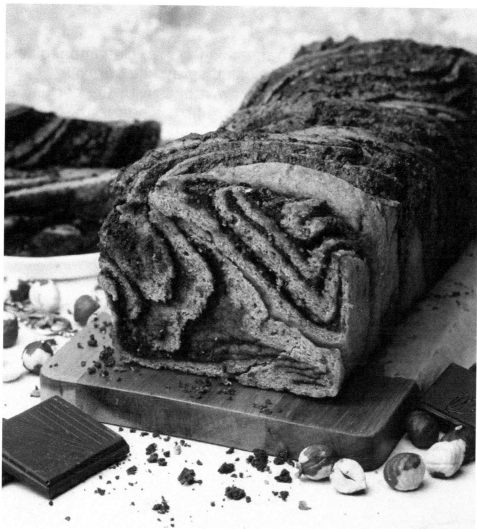

Preparation time: 10 minutes
Cooking time: 3 hours
Servings: 2

Ingredients:
- Cooking spray
- 1 cup almond flour
- ½ teaspoon baking soda
- ½ teaspoon cinnamon powder
- 1 tablespoon avocado oil
- 2 tablespoons maple syrup
- 2 eggs, whisked
- 1 tablespoon butter
- ½ tablespoon milk
- ½ teaspoon vanilla extract

- ½ cup dark chocolate, melted
- 2 tablespoons walnuts, chopped

Directions:
1. In a bowl, mix the flour with the baking soda, cinnamon, oil and the other ingredients except the cooking spray and stir well.
2. Grease a loaf pan that fits the slow cooker with the cooking spray, pour the bread batter into the pan, put the pan in the slow cooker after you've lined it with tin foil, put the lid on and cook on High for 3 hours.
3. Cool the sweet bread down, slice, divide between plates and serve for breakfast.

Nutrition: calories 200, fat 3, fiber 5, carbs 8, protein 4

Hash Brown Mix

Preparation time: 10 minutes
Cooking time: 3 hours
Servings: 6

Ingredients:
- 3 tablespoons butter
- ½ cup sour cream
- ¼ cup mushrooms, sliced
- ¼ teaspoon garlic powder
- ¼ cup yellow onion, chopped
- 1 cup milk
- 3 tablespoons flour
- 20 ounces hash browns
- Salt and black pepper to the taste
- 1 cup cheddar cheese, shredded
- Cooking spray

Directions:
1. Heat up a pan with the butter over medium-high heat, add mushrooms, onion and garlic powder, stir and cook for a few minutes.
2. Add flour and whisk well.
3. Add milk, stir really well and transfer everything to your Slow cooker greased with cooking spray.
4. Add hash browns, salt, pepper, sour cream and cheese, toss, cover and cook on High for 3 hours.
5. Divide between plates and serve for breakfast.

Nutrition: calories 262, fat 6, fiber 4, carbs 12, protein 6

Almond and Quinoa Bowls

Preparation time: 10 minutes
Cooking time: 5 hours
Servings: 2

Ingredients:
- 1 cup quinoa
- 2 cups almond milk
- 2 tablespoons butter, melted
- 2 tablespoons brown sugar
- A pinch of cinnamon powder
- A pinch of nutmeg, ground
- ¼ cup almonds, sliced
- Cooking spray

Directions:
1. Grease your slow cooker with the cooking spray, add the quinoa, milk, melted butter and the other ingredients, toss, put the lid on and cook on Low for 5 hours.
2. Divide the mix into bowls and serve for breakfast.

Nutrition: calories 211, fat 3, fiber 6, carbs 12, protein 5

Bacon and Egg Casserole

Preparation time: 10 minutes
Cooking time: 5 hours
Servings: 8

Ingredients:
- 20 ounces hash browns
- Cooking spray
- 8 ounces cheddar cheese, shredded
- 8 bacon slices, cooked and chopped
- 6 green onions, chopped
- ½ cup milk
- 12 eggs
- Salt and black pepper to the taste
- Salsa for serving

Directions:
1. Grease your Slow cooker with cooking spray, spread hash browns, cheese, bacon and green onions and toss.
2. In a bowl, mix the eggs with salt, pepper and milk and whisk really well.
3. Pour this over hash browns, cover and cook on Low for 5 hours.
4. Divide between plates and serve with salsa on top.

Nutrition: calories 300, fat 5, fiber 5, carbs 9, protein 5

Carrots Casserole

Preparation time: 10 minutes
Cooking time: 3 hours
Servings: 2

Ingredients:
- 1 teaspoon ginger, ground
- ½ pound carrots, peeled and grated
- 2 eggs, whisked
- ½ teaspoon garlic powder
- ½ teaspoon rosemary, dried
- Salt and black pepper to the taste
- 1 red onion, chopped
- 1 tablespoons parsley, chopped
- 2 garlic cloves, minced
- ½ tablespoon olive oil

Directions:
1. Grease your slow cooker with the oil and mix the carrots with the eggs, ginger and the other ingredients inside.
2. Toss, put the lid on, cook High for 3 hours, divide between plates and serve.

Nutrition: calories 218, fat 6, fiber 6, carbs 14, protein 5

Breakfast Rice Pudding

Preparation time: 10 minutes
Cooking time: 4 hours
Servings: 4

Ingredients:
- 1 cup coconut milk
- 2 cups water
- 1 cup almond milk
- ½ cup raisins
- 1 cup brown rice
- 2 teaspoons vanilla extract
- 2 tablespoons flaxseed
- 1 teaspoon cinnamon powder
- 2 tablespoons coconut sugar
- Cooking spray

Directions:
1. Grease your Slow cooker with the cooking spray, add coconut milk, water, almond milk, raisins, rice, vanilla, flaxseed and cinnamon, cover, cook on Low for 4 hours, stir, divide into bowls, sprinkle coconut sugar all over and serve.

Nutrition: calories 213, fat 3, fiber 6, carbs 10, protein 4

Cranberry Maple Oatmeal

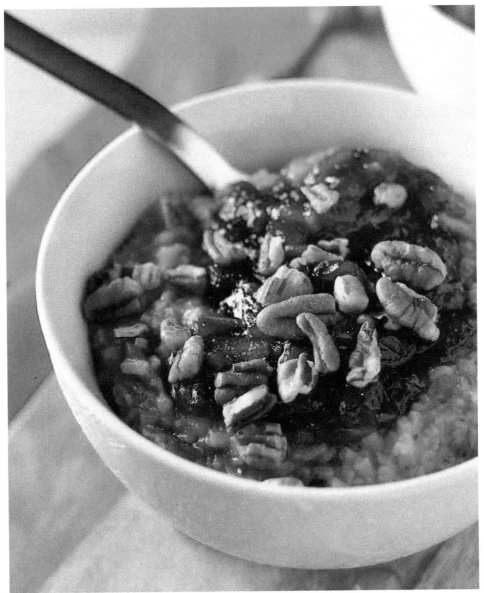

Preparation time: 10 minutes
Cooking time: 6 hours
Servings: 2

Ingredients:

- 1 cup almond milk
- ½ cup steel cut oats
- ½ cup cranberries
- ½ teaspoon vanilla extract
- 1 tablespoon maple syrup
- 1 tablespoon sugar

Directions:
1. In your slow cooker, mix the oats with the berries, milk and the other ingredients, toss, put the lid on and cook on Low for 6 hours.
2. Divide into bowls and serve for breakfast.

Nutrition: calories 200, fat 5, fiber 7, carbs 14, protein 4

Apple Breakfast Rice

Preparation time: 10 minutes
Cooking time: 7 hours
Servings: 4

Ingredients:
- 4 apples, cored, peeled and chopped
- 2 tablespoons butter
- 2 teaspoons cinnamon powder
- 1 and ½ cups brown rice
- ½ teaspoon vanilla extract
- A pinch of nutmeg, ground
- 5 cups milk

Directions:
1. Put the butter in your Slow cooker, add apples, cinnamon, rice, vanilla, nutmeg and milk, cover, cook on Low for 7 hours, stir, divide into bowls and serve for breakfast.

Nutrition: calories 214, fat 4, fiber 5, carbs 7, protein 4

Mushroom Casserole

Preparation time: 10 minutes
Cooking time: 5 hours
Servings: 2

Ingredients:
- ½ cup mozzarella, shredded
- 2 eggs, whisked
- ½ tablespoon balsamic vinegar
- ½ tablespoon olive oil
- 4 ounces baby kale
- 1 red onion, chopped
- ¼ teaspoon oregano
- ½ pound white mushrooms, sliced
- Salt and black pepper to the taste
- Cooking spray

Directions:
1. In a bowl, mix the eggs with the kale, mushrooms and the other ingredients except the cheese and cooking spray and stir well.
2. Grease your slow cooker with cooking spray, add the mushroom mix, spread, sprinkle the mozzarella all over, put the lid on and cook on Low for 5 hours.
3. Divide between plates and serve for breakfast.

Nutrition: calories 216, fat 6, fiber 8, carbs 12, protein 4

Quinoa and Banana Mix

Preparation time: 10 minutes
Cooking time: 6 hours
Servings: 8

Ingredients:
- 2 cups quinoa
- 2 bananas, mashed
- 4 cups water
- 2 cups blueberries
- 2 teaspoons vanilla extract
- 2 tablespoons maple syrup
- 1 teaspoon cinnamon powder
- Cooking spray

Directions:
1. Grease your Slow cooker with cooking spray, add quinoa, bananas, water, blueberries, vanilla, maple syrup and cinnamon, stir, cover and cook on Low for 6 hours.
2. Stir again, divide into bowls and serve for breakfast.

Nutrition: calories 200, fat 4, fiber 6, carbs 12, protein 4

Ginger Apple Bowls

Preparation time: 10 minutes
Cooking time: 6 hours
Servings: 2

Ingredients:
- 2 apples, cored, peeled and cut into medium chunks
- 1 tablespoon sugar
- 1 tablespoon ginger, grated
- 1 cup heavy cream
- ¼ teaspoon cinnamon powder
- ½ teaspoon vanilla extract
- ¼ teaspoon cardamom, ground

Directions:
1. In your slow cooker, combine the apples with the sugar, ginger and the other ingredients, toss, put the lid on and cook on Low for 6 hours.
2. Divide into bowls and serve for breakfast.

Nutrition: calories 201, fat 3, fiber 7, carbs 19, protein 4

Dates Quinoa

Preparation time: 10 minutes
Cooking time: 3 hours
Servings: 4

Ingredients:
- 1 cup quinoa
- 4 medjol dates, chopped
- 3 cups milk
- 1 apple, cored and chopped
- ¼ cup pepitas
- 2 teaspoons cinnamon powder
- 1 teaspoon vanilla extract
- ¼ teaspoon nutmeg, ground

Directions:
1. In your Slow cooker, mix quinoa with dates, milk, apple, pepitas, cinnamon, nutmeg and vanilla, stir, cover and cook on High for 3 hours.
2. Stir again, divide into bowls and serve.

Nutrition: calories 241, fat 4, fiber 4, carbs 10, protein 3

Granola Bowls

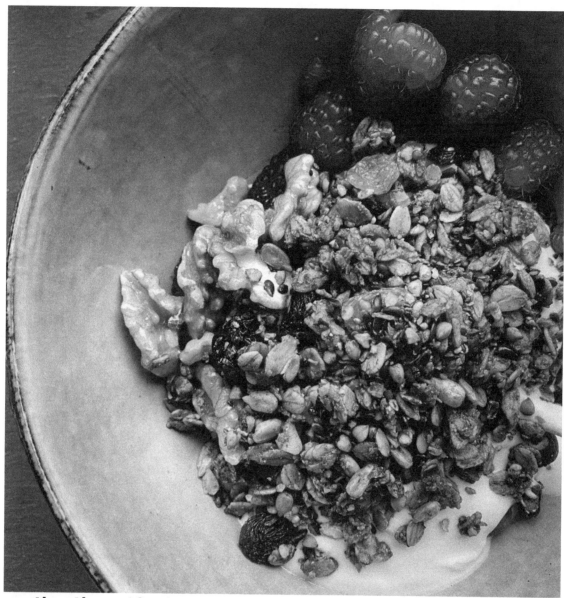

Preparation time: 10 minutes
Cooking time: 4 hours
Servings: 2

Ingredients:
- ½ cup granola
- ¼ cup coconut cream
- 2 tablespoons brown sugar
- 2 tablespoons cashew butter
- 1 teaspoon cinnamon powder
- ½ teaspoon nutmeg, ground

Directions:
1. In your slow cooker, mix the granola with the cream, sugar and the other ingredients, toss, put the lid on and cook on Low for 4 hours.
2. Divide into bowls and serve for breakfast.

Nutrition: calories 218, fat 6, fiber 9, carbs 17, protein 6

Cinnamon Quinoa

Preparation time: 10 minutes
Cooking time: 4 hours
Servings: 4

Ingredients:
- 1 cup quinoa
- 2 cups milk
- 2 cups water
- ¼ cup stevia
- 1 teaspoon cinnamon powder
- 1 teaspoon vanilla extract

Directions:
1. In your Slow cooker, mix quinoa with milk, water, stevia, cinnamon and vanilla, stir, cover, cook on Low for 3 hours and 30 minutes, stir, cook for 30 minutes more, divide into bowls and serve for breakfast.

Nutrition: calories 172, fat 4, fiber 3, carbs 8, protein 2

Squash Bowls

Preparation time: 10 minutes
Cooking time: 6 hours
Servings: 2

Ingredients:
- 2 tablespoons walnuts, chopped
- 2 cups squash, peeled and cubed
- ½ cup coconut cream
- ½ teaspoon cinnamon powder
- ½ tablespoon sugar

Directions:
1. In your slow cooker, mix the squash with the nuts and the other ingredients, toss, put the lid on and cook on Low for 6 hours.
2. Divide into bowls and serve.

Nutrition: calories 140, fat 1, fiber 2, carbs 2, protein 5

Quinoa and Apricots

Preparation time: 10 minutes
Cooking time: 10 hours
Servings: 6

Ingredients:
- ¾ cup quinoa
- ¾ cup steel cut oats
- 2 tablespoons honey
- 1 cup apricots, chopped
- 6 cups water
- 1 teaspoon vanilla extract
- ¾ cup hazelnuts, chopped

Directions:
1. In your Slow cooker, mix quinoa with oats honey, apricots, water, vanilla and hazelnuts, stir, cover and cook on Low for 10 hours.
2. Stir quinoa mix again, divide into bowls and serve for breakfast.

Nutrition: calories 200, fat 3, fiber 5, carbs 8, protein 6

Lamb and Eggs Mix

Preparation time: 10 minutes
Cooking time: 6 hours
Servings: 2

Ingredients:
- 1 pound lamb meat, ground
- 4 eggs, whisked
- 1 tablespoon basil, chopped
- ½ teaspoon cumin powder
- 1 tablespoon chili powder
- 1 red onion, chopped
- 1 tablespoon olive oil
- A pinch of salt and black pepper

Directions:
1. Grease the slow cooker with the oil and mix the lamb with the eggs, basil and the other ingredients inside.
2. Toss, put the lid on, cook on Low for 6 hours, divide into bowls and serve for breakfast.

Nutrition: calories 220, fat 2, fiber 2, carbs 6, protein 2

Blueberry Quinoa Oatmeal

Preparation time: 10 minutes
Cooking time: 8 hours
Servings: 4

Ingredients:
- ½ cup quinoa
- 1 cup steel cut oats
- 1 teaspoon vanilla extract
- 5 cups water
- Zest of 1 lemon, grated
- 1 teaspoon vanilla extract
- 2 tablespoons flaxseed
- 1 tablespoon butter, melted
- 3 tablespoons maple syrup
- 1 cup blueberries

Directions:
1. In your Slow cooker, mix butter with quinoa, water, oats, vanilla, lemon zest, flaxseed, maple syrup and blueberries, stir, cover and cook on Low for 8 hours.
2. Divide into bowls and serve for breakfast.

Nutrition: calories 189, fat 5, fiber 5, carbs 20, protein 5

Cauliflower Casserole

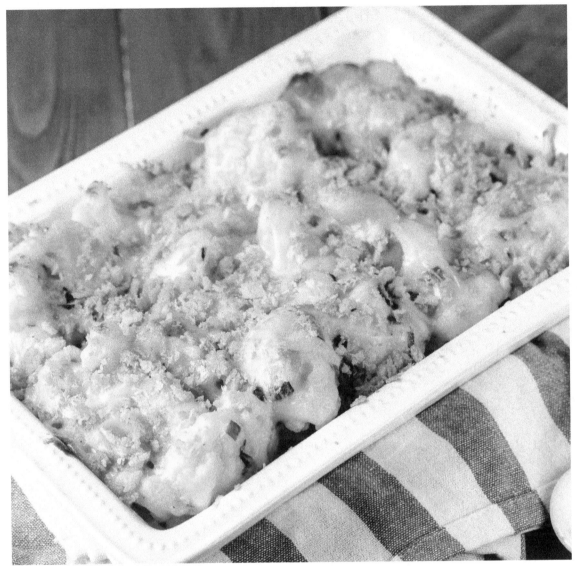

Preparation time: 10 minutes
Cooking time: 5 hours
Servings: 2

Ingredients:
- 1 pound cauliflower florets
- 3 eggs, whisked
- 1 red onion, sliced
- ½ teaspoon sweet paprika
- ½ teaspoon turmeric powder
- 1 garlic clove, minced
- A pinch of salt and black pepper
- Cooking spray

Directions:

1. Spray your slow cooker with the cooking spray, and mix the cauliflower with the eggs, onion and the other ingredients inside.
2. Put the lid on, cook on Low for 5 hours, divide between 2 plates and serve for breakfast.

Nutrition: calories 200, fat 3, fiber 6, carbs 13, protein 8

Lentils and Quinoa Mix

Preparation time: 10 minutes
Cooking time: 8 hours
Servings: 6

Ingredients:
- 3 garlic cloves, minced
- 1 yellow onion, chopped
- 1 celery stalk, chopped
- 2 red bell peppers, chopped
- 12 ounces canned tomatoes, chopped
- 4 cups veggie stock
- 1 cup lentils
- 14 ounces pinto beans
- 2 tablespoons chili powder
- ½ cup quinoa
- 1 tablespoons oregano, chopped
- 2 teaspoon cumin, ground

Directions:
1. In your Slow cooker, mix garlic with the onion, celery, bell peppers, tomatoes, stock, lentils, pinto beans, chili powder, quinoa, oregano and cumin, stir, cover, cook on Low for 8 hours, divide between plates and serve for breakfast

Nutrition: calories 231, fat 4, fiber 5, carbs 16, protein 4

Beef Meatloaf

Preparation time: 10 minutes
Cooking time: 4 hours
Servings: 2

Ingredients:
- 1 red onion, chopped
- 1 pound beef stew meat, ground
- ½ teaspoon chili powder
- 1 egg, whisked
- ½ teaspoon olive oil
- ½ teaspoon sweet paprika
- 2 tablespoons white flour
- ½ teaspoon oregano, chopped
- ½ tablespoon basil, chopped
- A pinch of salt and black pepper
- ½ teaspoon marjoram, dried

Directions:
1. In a bowl, mix the beef with the onion, chili powder and the other ingredients except the oil, stir well and shape your meatloaf.
2. Grease a loaf pan that fits your slow cooker with the oil, add meatloaf mix into the pan, put it in your slow cooker, put the lid on and cook on Low for 4 hours.
3. Slice and serve for breakfast.

Nutrition: calories 200, fat 6, fiber 12, carbs 17, protein 10

Butternut Squash Quinoa

Preparation time: 10 minutes
Cooking time: 6 hours
Servings: 6

Ingredients:
- 1 yellow onion, chopped
- 1 tablespoon olive oil
- 3 garlic cloves, minced
- 2 teaspoons oregano, dried
- 1 and ½ pound chicken breasts, skinless, boneless and chopped
- 2 teaspoons parsley, dried
- 2 teaspoons curry powder
- ½ teaspoon chili flakes
- Salt and black pepper to the taste
- 1 butternut squash, peeled and cubed
- 2/3 cup quinoa
- 12 ounces canned tomatoes, chopped
- 4 cups veggie stock

Directions:
1. In your Slow cooker, mix onion with oil, garlic, oregano, chicken, parsley, curry powder, chili, squash, quinoa, salt, pepper, tomatoes and stock, stir, cover and cook on Low for 6 hours.
2. Divide into bowls and serve for breakfast.

Nutrition: calories 231, fat 4, fiber 6, carbs 20, protein 5

Leek Casserole

Preparation time: 10 minutes
Cooking time: 4 hours
Servings: 2

Ingredients:
- 1 cup leek, chopped
- Cooking spray
- ½ cup mozzarella, shredded
- 1 garlic clove, minced
- 4 eggs, whisked
- 1 cup beef sausage, chopped
- 1 tablespoon cilantro, chopped

Directions:
1. Grease the slow cooker with the cooking spray and mix the leek with the mozzarella and the other ingredients inside.
2. Toss, spread into the pot, put the lid on and cook on Low for 4 hours.
3. Divide between plates and serve for breakfast.

Nutrition: calories 232, fat 4, fiber 8, carbs 17, protein 4

Chia Seeds Mix

Preparation time: 10 minutes
Cooking time: 8 hours
Servings: 4

Ingredients:
- 1 cup steel cut oats
- 1 cup water
- 3 cups almond milk
- 2 tablespoons chia seeds
- ¼ cup pomegranate seeds
- ¼ cup dried blueberries
- ¼ cup almonds, sliced

Directions:
1. In your Slow cooker, mix oats with water, almond milk, chia seeds, pomegranate ones, blueberries and almonds, stir, cover and cook on Low for 8 hours.
2. Stir again, divide into bowls and serve for breakfast.

Nutrition: calories 200, fat 3, fiber 7, carbs 16, protein 3

Eggs and Sweet Potato Mix

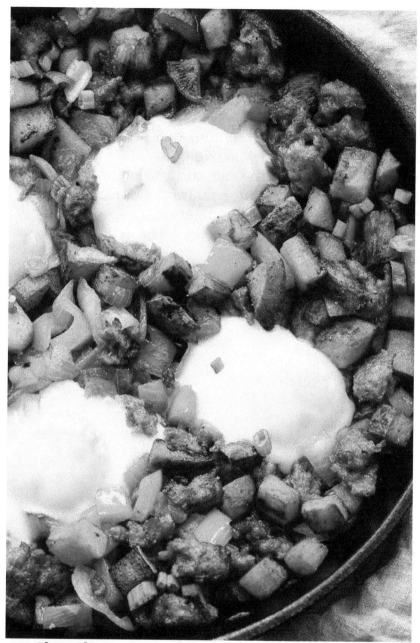

Preparation time: 10 minutes
Cooking time: 6 hours
Servings: 2

Ingredients:

- ½ red onion, chopped
- ½ green bell pepper, chopped
- 2 sweet potatoes, peeled and grated
- ½ red bell pepper, chopped

- 1 garlic clove, minced
- ½ teaspoon olive oil
- 4 eggs, whisked
- 1 tablespoon chives, chopped
- A pinch of red pepper, crushed
- A pinch of salt and black pepper

Directions:
1. In a bowl, mix the eggs with the onion, bell peppers and the other ingredients except the oil and whisk well.
2. Grease your slow cooker with the oil, add the eggs and potato mix, spread, put the lid on and cook on Low for 6 hours.
3. Divide everything between plates and serve.

Nutrition: calories 261, fat 6, fiber 6, carbs 16, protein 4

Chia Seeds and Chicken Breakfast

Preparation time: 10 minutes
Cooking time: 3 hours
Servings: 4

Ingredients:
- 1 pound chicken breasts, skinless, boneless and cubed
- ½ teaspoon basil, dried
- ¾ cup flaxseed, ground
- ¼ cup chia seeds
- ¼ cup parmesan, grated
- ½ teaspoon oregano, chopped
- Salt and black pepper to the taste
- 2 eggs
- 2 garlic cloves, minced

Directions:
1. In a bowl, mix flaxseed with chia seeds, parmesan, salt, pepper, oregano, garlic and basil and stir.
2. Put the eggs in a second bowl and whisk them well.
3. Dip chicken in eggs mix, then in chia seeds mix, put them in your Slow cooker after you've greased it with cooking spray, cover and cook on High for 3 hours.
4. Serve them right away for a Sunday breakfast.

Nutrition: calories 212, fat 3, fiber 4, carbs 17, protein 4

Pork and Eggplant Casserole

Preparation time: 10 minutes
Cooking time: 6 hours
Servings: 2

Ingredients:
- 1 red onion, chopped
- 1 eggplant, cubed
- ½ pound pork stew meat, ground
- 3 eggs, whisked
- ½ teaspoon chili powder
- ½ teaspoon garam masala
- 1 tablespoon sweet paprika
- 1 teaspoon olive oil

Directions:
1. In a bowl, mix the eggs with the meat, onion, eggplant and the other ingredients except the oil and stir well.
2. Grease your slow cooker with oil, add the pork and eggplant mix, spread into the pot, put the lid on and cook on Low for 6 hours.
3. Divide the mix between plates and serve for breakfast.

Nutrition: calories 261, fat 7, fiber 6, carbs 16, protein 7

Chocolate Quinoa

Preparation time: 10 minutes
Cooking time: 6 hours
Servings: 4

Ingredients:
- 1 cup quinoa
- 1 cup coconut milk
- 1 cup milk
- 2 tablespoons cocoa powder
- 3 tablespoons maple syrup
- 4 dark chocolate squares, chopped

Directions:
1. In your Slow cooker, mix quinoa with coconut milk, milk, cocoa powder, maple syrup and chocolate, stir, cover and cook on Low for 6 hours.
2. Stir quinoa mix again, divide into bowls and serve.

Nutrition: calories 215, fat 5, fiber 8, carbs 17, protein 4

Apple Spread

Preparation time: 10 minutes
Cooking time: 4 hours
Servings: 2

Ingredients:
- 2 apples, cored, peeled and pureed
- ½ cup coconut cream
- 2 tablespoons apple cider
- 2 tablespoons sugar
- ¼ teaspoon cinnamon powder
- ½ teaspoon lemon juice
- ¼ teaspoon ginger, grated

Directions:
1. In your slow cooker, mix the apple puree with the cream, sugar and the other ingredients, whisk, put the lid on and cook on High for 4 hours.
2. Blend using an immersion blender, cool down and serve for breakfast.

Nutrition: calories 172, fat 3, fiber 3, carbs 8, protein 3

Chai Breakfast Quinoa

Preparation time: 10 minutes
Cooking time: 6 hours
Servings: 2

Ingredients:
- 1 cup quinoa
- 1 egg white
- 2 cups milk
- ¼ teaspoon vanilla extract
- 1 and ½ tablespoons brown sugar
- ¼ teaspoon cardamom, ground
- ¼ teaspoon ginger, grated
- ¼ teaspoon cinnamon powder
- ¼ teaspoon vanilla extract
- ¼ teaspoon nutmeg, ground
- 1 tablespoons coconut flakes

Directions:
1. In your Slow cooker, mix quinoa with egg white, milk, vanilla, sugar, cardamom, ginger, cinnamon, vanilla and nutmeg, stir a bit, cover and cook on Low for 6 hours.
2. Stir, divide into bowls and serve for breakfast with coconut flakes on top.

Nutrition: calories 211, fat 4, fiber 6, carbs 10, protein 4

Cherries and Cocoa Oats

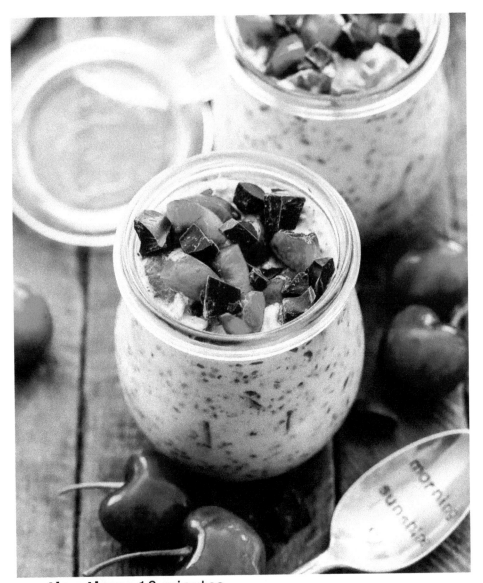

Preparation time: 10 minutes
Cooking time: 7 hours
Servings: 2

Ingredients:
- 1 cup almond milk
- ½ cup steel cut oats
- 1 tablespoon cocoa powder
- ½ cup cherries, pitted
- 2 tablespoons sugar
- ¼ teaspoon vanilla extract

Directions:

1. In your slow cooker, mix the almond milk with the cherries and the other ingredients, toss, put the lid on and cook on Low for 7 hours.
2. Divide into 2 bowls and serve for breakfast.

Nutrition: calories 150, fat 1, fiber 2, carbs 6, protein 5

Quinoa Breakfast Bake

Preparation time: 10 minutes
Cooking time: 7 hours
Servings: 4

Ingredients:
- 1 cup quinoa
- 4 tablespoons olive oil
- 2 cups water
- ½ cup dates, chopped
- 3 bananas, chopped
- ¼ cup coconut, shredded
- 2 teaspoons cinnamon powder
- 2 tablespoons brown sugar
- 1 cup walnuts, toasted and chopped

Directions:
1. Put the oil in your Slow cooker, add quinoa, water, dates, bananas, coconut, cinnamon, brown sugar and walnuts, stir, cover and cook on Low for 7 hours.
2. Divide into bowls and serve for breakfast.

Nutrition: calories 241, fat 4, fiber 8, carbs 16, protein 6

Beans Salad

Preparation time: 10 minutes
Cooking time: 6 hours
Servings: 2

Ingredients:
- 1 cup canned black beans, drained
- 1 cup canned red kidney beans, drained
- 1 cup baby spinach
- 2 spring onions, chopped
- ½ red bell pepper, chopped
- ¼ teaspoon turmeric powder
- ½ teaspoon garam masala
- ¼ cup veggie stock
- A pinch of cumin, ground
- A pinch of chili powder
- A pinch of salt and black pepper
- ½ cup salsa

Directions:
1. In your slow cooker, mix the beans with the spinach, onions and the other ingredients, toss, put the lid on and cook on High for 6 hours.
2. Divide the mix into bowls and serve for breakfast.

Nutrition: calories 130, fat 4, fiber 2, carbs 5, protein 4

Mocha Latte Quinoa Mix

Preparation time: 10 minutes
Cooking time: 6 hours
Servings: 4

Ingredients:
- 1 cup hot coffee
- 1 cup quinoa
- 1 cup coconut water
- ¼ cup chocolate chips
- ½ cup coconut cream

Directions:
1. In your Slow cooker, mix quinoa with coffee, coconut water and chocolate chips, cover and cook on Low for 6 hours.
2. Stir, divide into bowls, spread coconut cream all over and serve for breakfast.

Nutrition: calories 251, fat 4, fiber 7, carbs 15, protein 4

Peppers Rice Mix

Preparation time: 10 minutes
Cooking time: 3 hours
Servings: 2

Ingredients:
- ½ cup brown rice
- 1 cup chicken stock
- 2 spring onions, chopped
- ½ orange bell pepper, chopped
- ½ red bell pepper, chopped
- ½ green bell pepper, chopped
- 2 ounces canned green chilies, chopped
- ½ cup canned black beans, drained
- ½ cup mild salsa
- ½ teaspoon sweet paprika
- ½ teaspoon lime zest, grated
- A pinch of salt and black pepper

Directions:
1. In your slow cooker, mix the rice with the stock, spring onions and the other ingredients, toss, put the lid on and cook on High for 3 hours.
2. Divide the mix into bowls and serve for breakfast.

Nutrition: calories 140, fat 2, fiber 2, carbs 5, protein 5

Breakfast Butterscotch Pudding

Preparation time: 10 minutes
Cooking time: 1 hour and 40 minutes
Servings: 6

Ingredients:
- 4 ounces butter, melted
- 2 ounces brown sugar
- 7 ounces flour
- ¼ pint milk
- 1 teaspoon vanilla extract
- Zest of ½ lemon, grated
- 2 tablespoons maple syrup
- Cooking spray
- 1 egg

Directions:
1. In a bowl, mix butter with sugar, milk, vanilla, lemon zest, maple syrup and eggs and whisk well.
2. Add flour and whisk really well again.
3. Grease your Slow cooker with cooking spray, add pudding mix, spread, cover and cook on High for 1 hour and 30 minutes.
4. Divide between plates and serve for breakfast.

Nutrition: calories 271, fat 5, fiber 5, carbs 17, protein 4

Cashew Butter

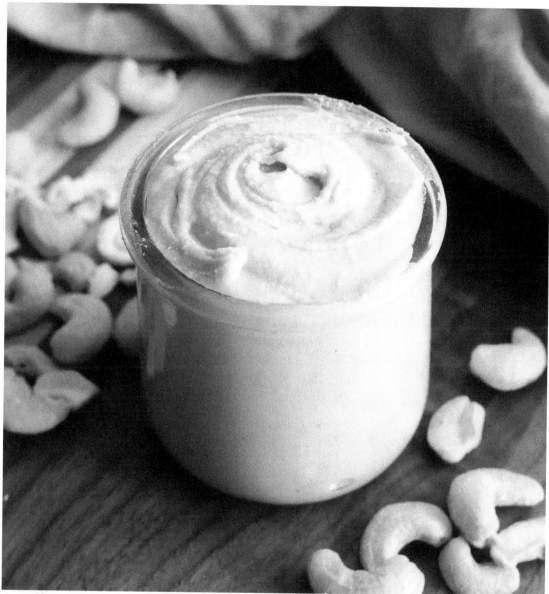

Preparation time: 10 minutes
Cooking time: 4 hours
Servings: 2

Ingredients:
- 1 cup cashews, soaked overnight, drained and blended
- ½ cup coconut cream
- ¼ teaspoon cinnamon powder
- 1 teaspoon lemon zest, grated
- 2 tablespoons sugar
- A pinch of ginger, ground

Directions:

1. In your slow cooker, mix the cashews with the cream and the other ingredients, whisk, put the lid on and cook on High for 4 hours.
2. Blend using an immersion blender, divide into jars, and serve for breakfast cold.

Nutrition: calories 143, fat 2, fiber 3, carbs 3, protein 4

French Breakfast Pudding

Preparation time: 10 minutes
Cooking time: 1 hour and 30 minutes
Servings: 4

Ingredients:
- 3 egg yolks
- 6 ounces double cream
- 1 teaspoon vanilla extract
- 2 tablespoons caster sugar

Directions:
1. In a bowl, mix the egg yolks with sugar and whisk well.
2. Add cream and vanilla extract, whisk well, pour into your 4 ramekins, place them in your Slow cooker, add some water to the slow cooker, cover and cook on High for 1 hour and 30 minutes.
3. Leave aside to cool down and serve.

Nutrition: calories 261, fat 5, fiber 6, carbs 15, protein 2

Pumpkin and Berries Bowls

Preparation time: 10 minutes
Cooking time: 4 hours
Servings: 2

Ingredients:
- ½ cup coconut cream
- 1 and ½ cups pumpkin, peeled and cubed
- 1 cup blackberries
- 2 tablespoons maple syrup
- ¼ teaspoon nutmeg, ground
- ½ teaspoon vanilla extract

Directions:
1. In your slow cooker, combine the pumpkin with the berries, cream and the other ingredients, toss, put the lid on and cook on Low for 4 hours.
2. Divide into bowls and serve for breakfast!

Nutrition: calories 120, fat 2, fiber 2, carbs 4, protein 2

Eggs and Sausage Casserole

Preparation time: 10 minutes
Cooking time: 8 hours
Servings: 4

Ingredients:

- 8 eggs, whisked
- 1 yellow onion, chopped
- 1 pound pork sausage, chopped
- 2 teaspoons basil, dried
- 1 tablespoon garlic powder
- Salt and black pepper to the taste
- 1 yellow bell pepper, chopped
- 1 teaspoon olive oil

Directions:

1. Grease your Slow cooker with the olive oil, add eggs, onion, pork sausage, basil, garlic powder, salt, pepper and yellow bell pepper, toss, cover and cook on Low for 8 hours.
2. Slice, divide between plates and serve for breakfast.

Nutrition: calories 301, fat 4, fiber 4, carbs 14, protein 7

Quinoa and Chia Pudding

Preparation time: 10 minutes
Cooking time: 6 hours
Servings: 2

Ingredients:
- 1 cup coconut cream
- 2 tablespoons chia seeds
- ½ cup almond milk
- 1 tablespoon sugar
- ½ cup quinoa, rinsed
- ½ teaspoon vanilla extract

Directions:
1. In your slow cooker, mix the cream with the chia seeds and the other ingredients, toss, put the lid on and cook on Low for 6 hours.
2. Divide into 2 bowls and serve for breakfast.

Nutrition: calories 120, fat 2, fiber 1, carbs 6, protein 4

Cauliflower Rice Pudding

Preparation time: 10 minutes
Cooking time: 2 hours
Servings: 2

Ingredients:
- ¼ cup maple syrup
- 3 cups almond milk
- 1 cup cauliflower rice
- 2 tablespoons vanilla extract

Directions:
1. Put cauliflower rice in your Slow cooker, add maple syrup, almond milk and vanilla extract, stir, cover and cook on High for 2 hours.
2. Stir your pudding again, divide into bowls and serve for breakfast.

Nutrition: calories 240, fat 2, fiber 2, carbs 15, protein 5

Beans Breakfast Bowls

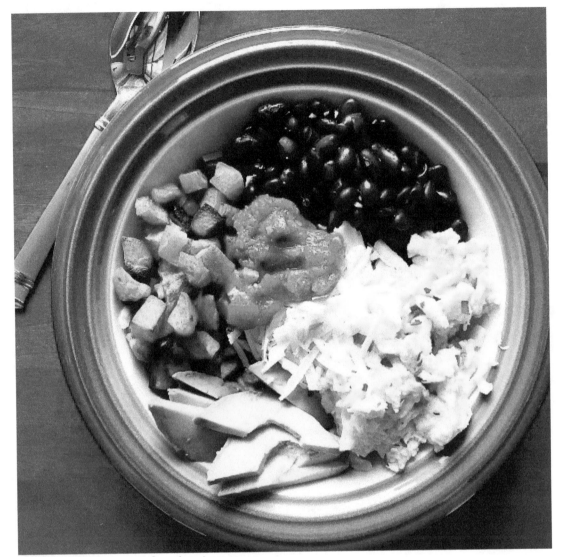

Preparation time: 10 minutes
Cooking time: 3 hours and 10 minutes
Servings: 2

Ingredients:
- 2 spring onions, chopped
- ½ green bell pepper, chopped
- ½ red bell pepper, chopped
- ½ yellow onion, chopped
- 5 ounces canned black beans, drained
- 5 ounces canned red kidney beans, drained
- 5 ounces canned pinto beans, drained
- ½ cup corn
- ½ teaspoon turmeric powder

- 1 teaspoons chili powder
- ½ teaspoon hot sauce
- A pinch of salt and black pepper
- 1 tablespoon olive oil

Directions:
1. Heat up a pan with the oil over medium-high heat, add the spring onions, bell peppers and the onion, sauté for 10 minutes and transfer to the slow cooker.
2. Add the beans and the other ingredients, toss, put the lid on and cook on High for 3 hours.
3. Divide the mix into bowls and serve for breakfast.

Nutrition: calories 240, fat 4, fiber 2, carbs 6, protein 9

Veggies Casserole

Preparation time: 10 minutes
Cooking time: 4 hours
Servings: 8

Ingredients:
- 8 eggs
- 4 egg whites
- 2 teaspoons mustard
- ¾ cup almond milk
- A pinch of salt and black pepper
- 2 red bell peppers, chopped
- 1 yellow onion, chopped
- 1 teaspoon sweet paprika
- 4 bacon strips, chopped
- 6 ounces cheddar cheese, shredded
- Cooking spray

Directions:
1. In a bowl, mix the eggs with egg whites, mustard, milk, salt, pepper and sweet paprika and whisk well.
2. Grease your Slow cooker with cooking spray and spread bell peppers, bacon and onion on the bottom.
3. Add mixed eggs, sprinkle cheddar all over, cover and cook on Low for 4 hours.
4. Divide between plates and serve for breakfast.

Nutrition: calories 262, fat 6, fiber 3, carbs 15, protein 7

Basil Sausage and Broccoli Mix

Preparation time: 10 minutes
Cooking time: 8 hours and 10 minutes
Servings: 2

Ingredients:
- 4 eggs, whisked
- 1 yellow onion, chopped
- 2 spring onions, chopped
- 1 cup pork sausage, chopped
- 1 cup broccoli florets
- 2 teaspoons basil, dried
- A pinch of salt and black pepper
- A drizzle of olive oil

Directions:
3. Heat up a pan with the oil over medium-high heat, add the yellow onion and the sausage, toss, cook for 10 minutes and transfer to the slow cooker.
4. Add the eggs and the other ingredients, toss, put the lid on and cook on Low for 8 hours.
5. Divide between plates and serve for breakfast.

Nutrition: calories 251, fat 4, fiber 4, carbs 6, protein 7

Arugula Frittata

Preparation time: 10 minutes
Cooking time: 4 hours
Servings: 4

Ingredients:
- 8 eggs
- Salt and black pepper to the taste
- ½ cup milk
- 1 teaspoon oregano, dried
- 4 cups baby arugula
- 1 and ¼ cup roasted red peppers, chopped
- ½ cup red onion, chopped
- ¾ cup goat cheese, crumbled
- Cooking spray

Directions:
1. In a bowl, mix the eggs with milk, oregano, salt and pepper and whisk well.
2. Grease your Slow cooker with cooking spray and spread roasted peppers, onion and arugula.
3. Add eggs mix, sprinkle goat cheese all over, cover, cook on Low for 4 hours, divide frittata between plates and serve for breakfast.

Nutrition: calories 269, fat 3, fiber 6, carbs 15, protein 4

Zucchini and Cauliflower Eggs Mix

Preparation time: 10 minutes
Cooking time: 6 hours
Servings: 2

Ingredients:
- 2 spring onions, chopped
- A pinch of salt and black pepper
- 4 eggs, whisked
- ½ cup cauliflower florets
- 1 zucchini, grated
- ¼ cup cheddar cheese, shredded
- ¼ cup whipping cream
- 1 tablespoon chives, chopped
- Cooking spray

Directions:
1. Grease the slow cooker with the cooking spray and mix the eggs with the spring onions, cauliflower and the other ingredients inside.
2. Put the lid on and cook on Low for 6 hours.
3. Divide the mix between plates and serve for breakfast.

Nutrition: calories 211, fat 7, fiber 4, carbs 5, protein 5

Mixed Egg and Sausage Scramble

Preparation time: 10 minutes
Cooking time: 6 hours
Servings: 6

Ingredients:
- 12 eggs
- 14 ounces sausages, sliced
- 1 cup milk
- 16 ounces cheddar cheese, shredded
- A pinch of salt and black pepper
- 1 teaspoon basil, dried
- 1 teaspoon oregano, dried
- Cooking spray

Directions:
1. Grease your Slow cooker with cooking spray, spread sausages on the bottom, crack eggs, add milk, basil, oregano, salt and pepper, whisk a bit, sprinkle cheddar all over, cover and cook on Low for 6 hours.
2. Divide egg and sausage scramble between plates and serve.

Nutrition: calories 267, fat 4, fiber 5, carbs 12, protein 9

Mushroom Quiche

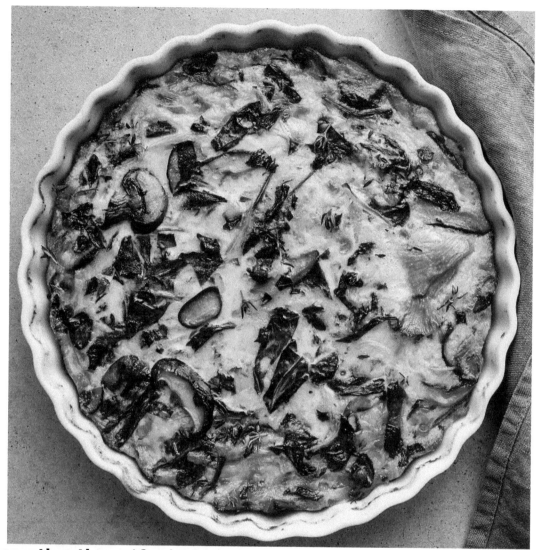

Preparation time: 10 minutes
Cooking time: 6 hours
Servings: 2

Ingredients:
- 2 cups baby Bella mushrooms, chopped
- ½ cup cheddar cheese, shredded
- 4 eggs, whisked
- ½ cup heavy cream
- 1 tablespoon basil, chopped
- 2 tablespoons chives, chopped
- A pinch of salt and black pepper
- ½ cup almond flour
- ¼ teaspoons baking soda

- Cooking spray

Directions:
1. In a bowl, mix the eggs with the cream, flour and the other ingredients except the cooking spray and stir well.
2. Grease the slow cooker with the cooking spray, pour the quiche mix, spread well, put the lid on and cook on High for 6 hours.
3. Slice the quiche, divide between plates and serve for breakfast.

Nutrition: calories 211, fat 6, fiber 6, carbs 6, protein 10

Worcestershire Asparagus Casserole

Preparation time: 10 minutes
Cooking time: 5 hours
Servings: 4

Ingredients:
- 2 pounds asparagus spears, cut into 1-inch pieces
- 1 cup mushrooms, sliced
- 1 teaspoon olive oil
- Salt and black pepper to the taste
- 2 cups coconut milk
- 1 teaspoon Worcestershire sauce
- 5 eggs, whisked

Directions:
1. Grease your Slow cooker with the oil and spread asparagus and mushrooms on the bottom.
2. In a bowl, mix the eggs with milk, salt, pepper and Worcestershire sauce, whisk, pour into the slow cooker, toss everything, cover and cook on Low for 6 hours.
3. Divide between plates and serve right away for breakfast.

Nutrition: calories 211, fat 4, fiber 4, carbs 8, protein 5

Scallions Quinoa and Carrots Bowls

Preparation time: 10 minutes
Cooking time: 4 hours
Servings: 2

Ingredients:
- 1 cup quinoa
- 2 cups veggie stock
- 4 scallions, chopped
- 2 carrots, peeled and grated
- 1 tablespoon olive oil
- A pinch of salt and black pepper
- 3 eggs, whisked
- 2 tablespoons cheddar cheese, grated
- 2 tablespoons heavy cream

Directions:
1. In a bowl mix the eggs with the cream, cheddar, salt and pepper and whisk.
2. Grease the slow cooker with the oil, add the quinoa, scallions, carrots and the stock, stir, put the lid on and cook on Low for 2 hours.
3. Add the eggs mix, stir the whole thing, cook on Low for 2 more hours, divide into bowls and serve for breakfast.

Nutrition: calories 172, fat 5, fiber 4, carbs 6, protein 8

Peppers, Kale and Cheese Omelet

Preparation time: 10 minutes
Cooking time: 3 hours
Servings: 4

Ingredients:
- 1 teaspoon olive oil
- 7 ounces roasted red peppers, chopped
- 6 ounces baby kale
- Salt and black pepper to the taste
- 6 ounces feta cheese, crumbled
- ¼ cup green onions, sliced
- 7 eggs, whisked

Directions:
1. In a bowl, mix the eggs with cheese, kale, red peppers, green onions, salt and pepper, whisk well, pour into the Slow cooker after you've greased it with the oil, cover, cook on Low for 3 hours, divide between plates and serve right away.

Nutrition: calories 231, fat 7, fiber 4, carbs 7, protein 14

Ham Omelet

Preparation time: 10 minutes
Cooking time: 3 hours
Servings: 2

Ingredients:
- Cooking spray
- 4 eggs, whisked
- 1 tablespoon sour cream
- 2 spring onions, chopped
- 1 small yellow onion, chopped
- ½ cup ham, chopped
- ½ cup cheddar cheese, shredded
- 1 tablespoon chives, chopped
- A pinch of salt and black pepper

Directions:
1. Grease your slow cooker with the cooking spray and mix the eggs with the sour cream, spring onions and the other ingredients inside.
2. Toss the mix, spread into the pot, put the lid on and cook on High for 3 hours.
3. Divide the mix between plates and serve for breakfast right away.

Nutrition: calories 192, fat 6, fiber 5, carbs 6, protein 12

Salmon Frittata

Preparation time: 10 minutes
Cooking time: 3 hours and 40 minutes
Servings: 3

Ingredients:
- 4 eggs, whisked
- ½ teaspoon olive oil
- 2 tablespoons green onions, chopped
- Salt and black pepper to the taste
- 4 ounces smoked salmon, chopped

Directions:
1. Drizzle the oil in your Slow cooker, add eggs, salt and pepper, whisk, cover and cook on Low for 3 hours.
2. Add salmon and green onions, toss a bit, cover, cook on Low for 40 minutes more and divide between plates.
3. Serve right away for breakfast.

Nutrition: calories 220, fat 10, fiber 2, carbs 15, protein 7

Peppers and Eggs Mix

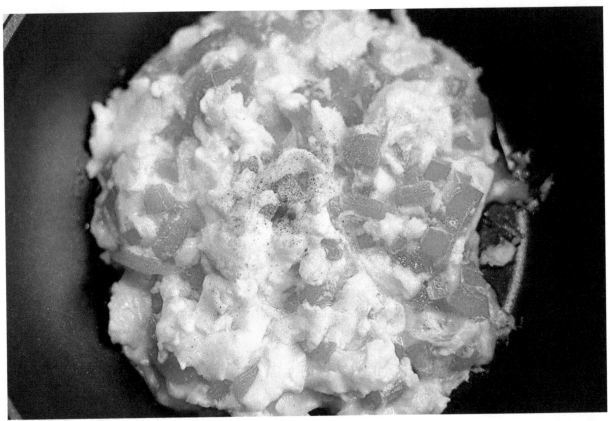

Preparation time: 10 minutes
Cooking time: 4 hours
Servings: 2

Ingredients:
- 4 eggs, whisked
- ½ teaspoon coriander, ground
- ½ teaspoon rosemary, dried
- 2 spring onions, chopped
- 1 red bell pepper, cut into strips
- 1 green bell pepper, cut into strips
- 1 yellow bell pepper, cut into strips
- ¼ cup heavy cream
- ½ teaspoon garlic powder
- A pinch of salt and black pepper
- 1 teaspoon sweet paprika
- Cooking spray

Directions:
5. Grease your slow cooker with the cooking spray, and mix the eggs with the coriander, rosemary and the other ingredients into the pot.

6. Put the lid on, cook on Low for 4 hours, divide between plates and serve for breakfast.

Nutrition: calories 172, fat 6, fiber 3, carbs 6, protein 7

Creamy Breakfast

Preparation time: 5 minutes
Cooking time: 3 hours
Servings: 1

Ingredients:
- 1 teaspoon cinnamon powder
- ½ teaspoon nutmeg, ground
- ½ cup almonds, chopped
- 1 teaspoon sugar
- 1 and ½ cup heavy cream
- ¼ teaspoon cardamom, ground
- ¼ teaspoon cloves, ground

Directions:
1. In your Slow cooker, mix cream with cinnamon, nutmeg, almonds, sugar, cardamom and cloves, stir, cover, cook on Low for 3 hours, divide into bowls and serve for breakfast

Nutrition: calories 250, fat 12, fiber 4, carbs 8, protein 16

Baby Spinach Rice Mix

Preparation time: 10 minutes
Cooking time: 6 hours
Servings: 4

Ingredients:
- ¼ cup mozzarella, shredded
- ½ cup baby spinach
- ½ cup wild rice
- 1 and ½ cups chicken stock
- ½ teaspoon turmeric powder
- ½ teaspoon oregano, dried
- A pinch of salt and black pepper
- 3 scallions, minced
- ¾ cup goat cheese, crumbled

Directions:
4. In your slow cooker, mix the rice with the stock, turmeric and the other ingredients, toss, put the lid on and cook on Low for 6 hours.
5. Divide the mix into bowls and serve for breakfast.

Nutrition: calories 165, fat 1.2, fiber 3.5, carbs 32.6, protein 7.6

Brussels Sprouts Omelet

Preparation time: 10 minutes
Cooking time: 4 hours
Servings: 4

Ingredients:
- 4 eggs, whisked
- Salt and black pepper to the taste
- 1 tablespoon olive oil
- 2 green onions, minced
- 2 garlic cloves, minced
- 12 ounces Brussels sprouts, sliced
- 2 ounces bacon, chopped

Directions:
1. Drizzle the oil on the bottom of your Slow cooker and spread Brussels sprouts, garlic, bacon, green onions, eggs, salt and pepper, toss, cover and cook on Low for 4 hours.
2. Divide between plates and serve right away for breakfast.

Nutrition: calories 240, fat 7, fiber 4, carbs 7, protein 13

Herbed Egg Scramble

Preparation time: 10 minutes
Cooking time: 6 hours
Servings: 2

Ingredients:
- 4 eggs, whisked
- ¼ cup heavy cream
- ¼ cup mozzarella, shredded
- 1 tablespoon chives, chopped
- 1 tablespoon oregano, chopped
- 1 tablespoon rosemary, chopped
- A pinch of salt and black pepper
- Cooking spray

Directions:
3. Grease your slow cooker with the cooking spray, and mix the eggs with the cream, herbs and the other ingredients inside.
4. Stir well, put the lid on, cook for 6 hours on Low, stir once again, divide between plates and serve.

Nutrition: calories 203, fat 15.7, fiber 1.7, carbs 3.8, protein 12.8

Chicken Frittata

Preparation time: 10 minutes
Cooking time: 3 hours
Servings: 2

Ingredients:
- ½ cup chicken, cooked and shredded
- 1 teaspoon mustard
- 1 tablespoon mayonnaise
- 1 tomato, chopped
- 2 bacon slices, cooked and crumbled
- 4 eggs
- 1 small avocado, pitted, peeled and chopped
- Salt and black pepper to the taste

Directions:
1. In a bowl, mix the eggs with salt, pepper, chicken, avocado, tomato, bacon, mayo and mustard, toss, transfer to your Slow cooker, cover and cook on Low for 3 hours.
2. Divide between plates and serve for breakfast

Nutrition: calories 300, fat 32, fiber 6, carbs 15, protein 25

Peas and Rice Bowls

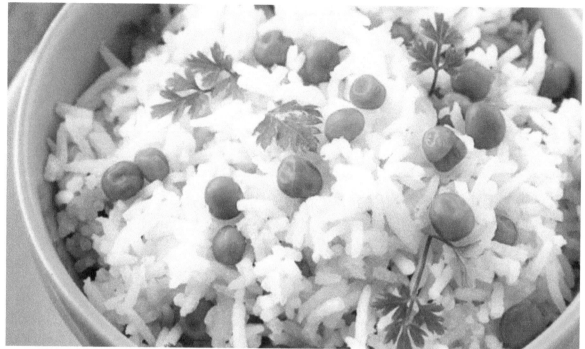

Preparation time: 10 minutes
Cooking time: 6 hours
Servings: 2

Ingredients:

- ¼ cup peas
- 1 cup wild rice
- 2 cups veggie stock
- ¼ cup heavy cream
- 1 tablespoon dill, chopped
- 3 spring onions, chopped
- ½ teaspoon coriander, ground
- ½ teaspoon allspice, ground
- A pinch of salt and black pepper
- ¼ cup cheddar cheese, shredded
- 1 teaspoon olive oil

Directions:

1. Grease the slow cooker with the oil, add the rice, peas, stock and the other ingredients except the dill and heavy cream, stir, put the lid on and cook on Low for 3 hours.
2. Add the remaining ingredients, stir the mix, put the lid back on, cook on Low for 3 more hours, divide into bowls and serve for breakfast.

Nutrition: calories 442, fat 13.6, fiber 6.8, carbs 66, protein 17.4

Mushrooms Casserole

Preparation time: 10 minutes
Cooking time: 4 hours
Servings: 4

Ingredients:
- 1 teaspoon lemon zest, grated
- 10 ounces goat cheese, cubed
- 1 tablespoon lemon juice
- 1 tablespoon apple cider vinegar
- 1 tablespoon olive oil
- 2 garlic cloves, minced
- 10 ounces spinach, torn
- ½ cup yellow onion, chopped
- ½ teaspoon basil, dried
- 8 ounces mushrooms, sliced
- Salt and black pepper to the taste
- Cooking spray

Directions:
4. Spray your Slow cooker with cooking spray, arrange cheese cubes on the bottom and add lemon zest, lemon juice, vinegar, olive oil, garlic, spinach, onion, basil, mushrooms, salt and pepper.
5. Toss well, cover, cook on Low for 4 hours, divide between plates and serve for breakfast right away.

Nutrition: calories 276, fat 6, fiber 5, carbs 7, protein 4

Asparagus Casserole

Preparation time: 10 minutes
Cooking time: 5 hours
Servings: 2

Ingredients:
- 1 pound asparagus spears, cut into medium pieces
- 1 red onion, sliced
- 4 eggs, whisked
- ½ cup cheddar cheese, shredded
- ¼ cup heavy cream
- 1 tablespoon chives, chopped
- A drizzle of olive oil
- A pinch of salt and black pepper

Directions:
4. Grease your slow cooker with the oil, and mix the eggs with the asparagus, onion and the other ingredients except the cheese into the pot.
5. Sprinkle the cheese all over, put the lid on and cook on Low for 5 hours.
6. Divide between plates and serve right away for breakfast.

Nutrition: calories 359, fat 24, fiber 6, carbs 15.5, protein 24.1

Carrot Pudding

Preparation time: 10 minutes
Cooking time: 8 hours
Servings: 4

Ingredients:
- 4 carrots, grated
- 1 and ½ cups milk
- A pinch of nutmeg, ground
- A pinch of cloves, ground
- ½ teaspoon cinnamon powder
- 2 tablespoons maple syrup
- ¼ cup walnuts, chopped
- 1 teaspoon vanilla extract

Directions:
1. In your Slow cooker, mix carrots with milk, cloves, nutmeg, cinnamon, maple syrup, walnuts and vanilla extract, stir, cover and cook on Low for 8 hours.
2. Divide into bowls and serve for breakfast.

Nutrition: calories 215, fat 4, fiber 4, carbs 7, protein 7

Slow Cooker Lunch Recipes

Turkey Lunch

Preparation time: 10 minutes
Cooking time: 4 hours and 20 minutes
Servings: 12

Ingredients:
- ½ teaspoon thyme, dried
- ½ teaspoon garlic powder
- Salt and black pepper to the taste
- 2 turkey breast halves, boneless
- 1/3 cup water
- 1 cup grape juice
- 2 cups raspberries
- 2 apples, peeled and chopped
- 2 cups blueberries
- A pinch of red pepper flakes, crushed
- ¼ teaspoon ginger powder

Directions:
1. In your Slow cooker, mix water with salt, pepper, thyme and garlic powder and stir.
2. Add turkey breast halves, toss, cover and cook on Low for 4 hours.
3. Meanwhile, heat up a pan over medium-high heat, add grape juice, apples, raspberries, blueberries, pepper flakes and ginger, stir, bring to a simmer, cook for 20 minutes and take off heat.
4. Divide turkey between plates, drizzle berry sauce all over and serve for lunch.

Nutrition: calories 215, fat 2, fiber 3, carbs 12, protein 26

Seafood Soup

Preparation time: 10 minutes
Cooking time: 8 hours
Servings: 2

Ingredients:
- 2 cups chicken stock
- 1 cup coconut milk
- 1 sweet potato, cubed
- ½ yellow onion, chopped
- 1 bay leaf
- 1 carrot, peeled and sliced
- ½ tablespoon thyme, dried
- Salt and black pepper to the taste
- ½ pounds salmon fillets, skinless, boneless cubed
- 12 shrimp, peeled and deveined
- 1 tablespoon chives, chopped

Directions:
1. In your slow cooker, mix the carrot with the sweet potato, onion and the other ingredients except the salmon, shrimp and chives, toss, put the lid on and cook on Low for 6 hours.
2. Add the rest of the ingredients, toss, put the lid on and cook on Low for 2 more hours.
3. Divide the soup into bowls and serve for lunch.

Nutrition: calories 354, fat 10, fiber 4, carbs 17, protein 12

Lunch Roast

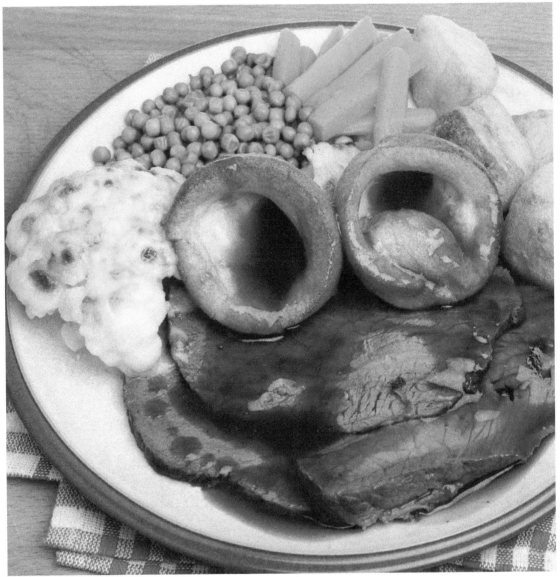

Preparation time: 10 minutes
Cooking time: 8 hours
Servings: 8

Ingredients:
- 2 pounds beef chuck roast
- Salt and black pepper to the taste
- 1 yellow onion, chopped
- 2 teaspoons olive oil
- 8 ounces tomato sauce
- ¼ cup lemon juice
- ¼ cup water
- ¼ cup ketchup

- ¼ cup apple cider vinegar
- 1 tablespoons Worcestershire sauce
- 2 tablespoons brown sugar
- ½ teaspoon mustard powder
- ½ teaspoons paprika

Directions:

1. In your Slow cooker, mix beef with salt, pepper, onion oil, tomato sauce, lemon juice, water, ketchup, vinegar, Worcestershire sauce, sugar, mustard and paprika, toss well, cover and cook on Low for 8 hours.
2. Slice roast, divide between plates, drizzle cooking sauce all over and serve for lunch.

Nutrition: calories 243, fat 12, fiber 2, carbs 10, protein 23

Sesame Salmon Bowls

Preparation time: 10 minutes
Cooking time: 3 hours
Servings: 2

Ingredients:
- 2 salmon fillets, boneless and roughly cubed
- 1 cup cherry tomatoes, halved
- 3 spring onions, chopped
- 1 cup baby spinach
- ½ cup chicken stock
- Salt and black pepper to the taste
- 2 tablespoons balsamic vinegar
- 2 tablespoons lemon juice
- 1 teaspoon sesame seeds

Directions:
1. In your slow cooker, mix the salmon with the cherry tomatoes, spring onions and the other ingredients, toss gently, put the lid on and cook on Low for 3 hours.
2. Divide everything into bowls and serve.

Nutrition: calories 230, fat 4, fiber 2, carbs 7, protein 6

Fajitas

Preparation time: 10 minutes
Cooking time: 3 hours
Servings: 8

Ingredients:
- 1 and ½ pounds beef sirloin, cut into thin strips
- 2 tablespoons lemon juice
- 2 tablespoons olive oil
- 1 garlic clove, minced
- 1 and ½ teaspoon cumin, ground
- Salt and black pepper to the taste
- ½ teaspoon chili powder
- A pinch of red pepper flakes, crushed
- 1 red bell pepper, cut into thin strips
- 1 yellow onion, cut into thin strips
- 8 mini tortillas

Directions:
1. Heat up a pan with the oil over medium-high heat, add beef strips, brown them for a few minutes and transfer to your Slow cooker.
2. Add lemon juice, garlic, cumin, salt, pepper, chili powder and pepper flakes to the slow cooker as well, cover and cook on High for 2 hours.
3. Add bell pepper and onion, stir and cook on High for 1 more hour.
4. Divide beef mix between your mini tortillas and serve for lunch.

Nutrition: calories 220, fat 9, fiber 2, carbs 14, protein 20

Shrimp Stew

Preparation time: 10 minutes
Cooking time: 3 hours
Servings: 2

Ingredients:
- 1 garlic clove, minced
- 1 red onion, chopped
- 1 cup canned tomatoes, crushed
- 1 cup veggie stock
- ½ teaspoon turmeric powder
- 1 pound shrimp, peeled and deveined
- ½ teaspoon coriander, ground
- ½ teaspoon thyme, dried
- ½ teaspoon basil, dried
- A pinch of salt and black pepper
- A pinch of red pepper flakes

Directions:
1. In your slow cooker, mix the onion with the garlic, shrimp and the other ingredients, toss, put the lid on and cook on High for 3 hours.
2. Divide the stew into bowls and serve.

Nutrition: calories 313, fat 4.2, fiber 2.5, carbs 13.2, protein 53.3

Teriyaki Pork

Preparation time: 10 minutes
Cooking time: 7 hours
Servings: 8

Ingredients:
- 2 tablespoons sugar
- 2 tablespoons soy sauce
- ¾ cup apple juice
- 1 teaspoon ginger powder
- 1 tablespoon white vinegar
- Salt and black pepper to the taste
- ¼ teaspoon garlic powder
- 3 pounds pork loin roast, halved
- 7 teaspoons cornstarch
- 3 tablespoons water

Directions:
1. In your Slow cooker, mix apple juice with sugar, soy sauce, vinegar, ginger, garlic powder, salt, pepper and pork loin, toss well, cover and cook on Low for 7 hours.
2. Transfer cooking juices to a small pan, heat up over medium-high heat, add cornstarch mixed with water, stir well, cook for 2 minutes until it thickens and take off heat.
3. Slice roast, divide between plates, drizzle sauce all over and serve for lunch.

Nutrition: calories 247, fat 8, fiber 1, carbs 9, protein 33

Garlic Shrimp and Spinach

Preparation time: 10 minutes
Cooking time: 2 hours
Servings: 2

Ingredients:
- 1 pound shrimp, peeled and deveined
- 1 cup baby spinach
- ½ teaspoon sweet paprika
- ½ cup chicken stock
- 1 garlic clove, minced
- 2 jalapeno peppers, chopped
- Cooking spray
- 1 teaspoon coriander, ground
- ½ teaspoon rosemary, dried
- A pinch of sea salt and black pepper

Directions:
1. Grease the slow cooker with the oil, add the shrimp, spinach and the other ingredients, toss, put the lid on and cook on High for 2 hours.
2. Divide everything between plates and serve for lunch.

Nutrition: calories 200, fat 4, fiber 6, carbs 16, protein 4

Beef Stew

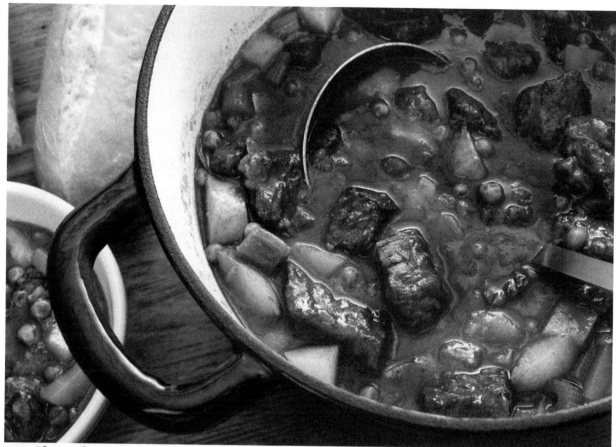

Preparation time: 10 minutes
Cooking time: 7 hours and 30 minutes
Servings: 5

Ingredients:
- 2 potatoes, peeled and cubed
- 1 pound beef stew meat, cubed
- 11 ounces tomato juice
- 14 ounces beef stock
- 2 celery ribs, chopped
- 2 carrots, chopped
- 3 bay leaves
- 1 yellow onion, chopped
- Salt and black pepper to the taste
- ½ teaspoon chili powder
- ½ teaspoon thyme, dried
- 1 tablespoon water
- 2 tablespoons cornstarch
- ½ cup peas

- ½ cup corn

Directions:
1. In your Slow cooker, mix potatoes with beef, tomato juice, stock, ribs, carrots, bay leaves, onion, salt, pepper, chili powder and thyme, stir, cover and cook on Low for 7 hours.
2. Add cornstarch mixed with water, peas and corn, stir, cover and cook on Low for 30 minutes more.
3. Divide into bowls and serve for lunch.

Nutrition: calories 273, fat 7, fiber 6, carbs 30, protein 22

Ginger Salmon

Preparation time: 10 minutes
Cooking time: 3 hours
Servings: 2

Ingredients:
- 2 salmon fillets, boneless
- 1 tablespoon olive oil
- 1 tablespoon balsamic vinegar
- 1 tablespoon ginger, grated
- A pinch of nutmeg, ground
- A pinch of cloves, ground
- A pinch of salt and black pepper
- 1 teaspoon onion powder
- ½ teaspoon cayenne pepper
- ¼ cup chicken stock

Directions:
1. Grease the slow cooker with the oil and arrange the salmon fillets inside.
2. Add the vinegar, ginger and the other ingredients, rub gently, put the lid on and cook on Low for 3 hours.
3. Divide the fish between plates and serve with a side salad for lunch.

Nutrition: calories 315, fat 18.4, fiber 0.6, carbs 3.6, protein 35.1

Apple and Onion Lunch Roast

Preparation time: 10 minutes
Cooking time: 5 hours
Servings: 8

Ingredients:

- 1 beef sirloin roast, halved
- Salt and black pepper to the taste
- 1 cup water
- ½ teaspoon soy sauce
- 1 apple, cored and quartered
- ¼ teaspoon garlic powder
- ½ teaspoon Worcestershire sauce
- 1 yellow onion, cut into medium wedges
- 2 tablespoons water
- 2 tablespoons cornstarch
- 1/8 teaspoon browning sauce
- Cooking spray

Directions:

1. Grease a pan with the cooking spray, heat it up over medium-high heat, add roast, brown it for a few minutes on each side and transfer to your Slow cooker.
2. Add salt, pepper, soy sauce, garlic powder, Worcestershire sauce, onion and apple, cover and cook on Low for 6 hours.
3. Transfer cooking juices from the slow cooker to a pan, heat it up over medium heat, add cornstarch, water and browning sauce, stir well, cook for a few minutes and take off heat.
4. Slice roast, divide between plates, drizzle sauce all over and serve for lunch.

Nutrition: calories 242, fat 8, fiber 1, carbs 8, protein 34

Creamy Cod Stew

Preparation time: 10 minutes
Cooking time: 3 hours
Servings: 2

Ingredients:
- ½ pound cod fillets, boneless and cubed
- 2 spring onions, chopped
- ¼ cup heavy cream
- 1 carrot, sliced
- 1 zucchini, cubed
- 1 tomato, cubed
- 1 cup chicken stock
- 1 tablespoon olive oil
- 1 green bell pepper, chopped
- 1 tablespoon chives, chopped
- A pinch of salt and black pepper

Directions:
1. In your slow cooker, combine the fish with the spring onions, carrot and the other ingredients except the cream, toss gently, put the lid on and cook on High for 2 hours and 30 minutes.
2. Add the cream, toss gently, put the lid back on, cook the stew on Low for 30 minutes more, divide into bowls and serve.

Nutrition: calories 175, fat 13.3, fiber 3.4, carbs 14, protein 3.3

Stuffed Peppers

Preparation time: 10 minutes
Cooking time: 4 hours
Servings: 4

Ingredients:
- 15 ounces canned black beans, drained
- 4 sweet red peppers, tops and seeds discarded
- 1 cup pepper jack cheese, shredded
- 1 yellow onion, chopped
- ¾ cup salsa
- ½ cup corn
- 1/3 cup white rice
- ½ teaspoon cumin, ground
- 1 and ½ teaspoons chili powder

Directions:
1. In a bowl, mix black beans with cheese, salsa, onion, corn, rice, cumin and chili powder and stir well.
2. Stuff peppers with this mix, place them in your Slow cooker, cover and cook on Low for 4 hours.
3. Divide between plates and serve them for lunch.

Nutrition: calories 317, fat 10, fiber 8, carbs 43, protein 12

Sweet Potato and Clam Chowder

Preparation time: 10 minutes
Cooking time: 3 hours and 30 minutes
Servings: 2

Ingredients:
- 1 small yellow onion, chopped
- 1 carrot, chopped
- 1 red bell pepper, cubed
- 6 ounces canned clams, chopped
- 1 sweet potato, chopped
- 2 cups chicken stock
- ½ cup coconut milk
- 1 teaspoon Worcestershire sauce

Directions:
1. In your slow cooker, mix the onion with the carrot, clams and the other ingredients, toss, put the lid on and cook on High for 3 hours.
2. Divide the chowder into bowls and serve for lunch.

Nutrition: calories 288, fat 15.3, fiber 5.9, carbs 36.4, protein 5

Beans and Pumpkin Chili

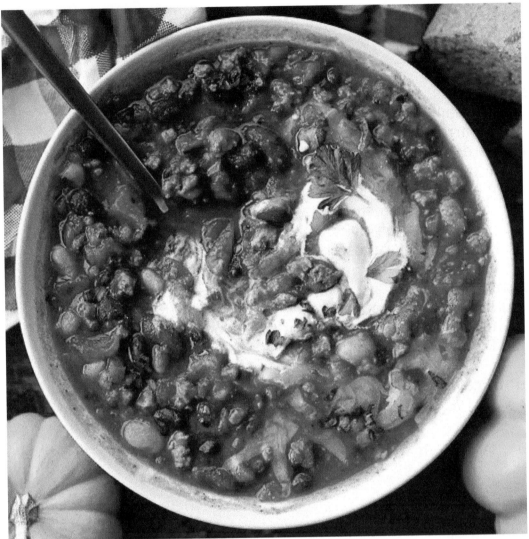

Preparation time: 10 minutes
Cooking time: 4 hours
Servings: 10

Ingredients:
- 1 yellow bell pepper, chopped
- 1 yellow onion, chopped
- 3 garlic cloves, minced
- 2 tablespoons olive oil
- 3 cups chicken stock
- 30 ounces canned black beans, drained
- 14 ounces pumpkin, cubed
- 2 and ½ cups turkey meat, cooked and cubed
- 2 teaspoons parsley, dried
- 1 and ½ teaspoon oregano, dried

- 2 teaspoons chili powder
- 1 and ½ teaspoon cumin, ground
- Salt and black pepper to the taste

Directions:

1. Heat up a pan with the oil over medium-high heat, add bell pepper, onion and garlic, stir, cook for a few minutes and transfer to your Slow cooker.
2. Add stock, beans, pumpkin, turkey, parsley, oregano, chili powder, cumin, salt and pepper, stir, cover and cook on Low for 4 hours.
3. Divide into bowls and serve right away for lunch.

Nutrition: calories 200, fat 5, fiber 7, carbs 20, protein 15

Maple Chicken Mix

Preparation time: 10 minutes
Cooking time: 6 hours
Servings: 2

Ingredients:
- 2 spring onions, chopped
- 1 pound chicken breast, skinless and boneless
- 2 garlic cloves, minced
- 1 tablespoon maple syrup
- A pinch of salt and black pepper
- ½ cup chicken stock
- ½ cup tomato sauce
- 1 tablespoon chives, chopped
- 1 teaspoon basil, dried

Directions:
1. In your slow cooker mix the chicken with the garlic, maple syrup and the other ingredients, toss, put the lid on and cook on Low for 6 hours.
2. Divide the mix between plates and serve for lunch.

Nutrition: calories 200, fat 3, fiber 3, carbs 17, protein 6

Chicken and Peppers Mix

Preparation time: 10 minutes
Cooking time: 4 hours
Servings: 6

Ingredients:
- 24 ounces tomato sauce
- ¼ cup parmesan, grated
- 1 yellow onion, chopped
- 2 garlic cloves, minced
- 1 teaspoon basil, dried
- 1 teaspoon oregano, dried
- Salt and black pepper to the taste
- 6 chicken breast halves, skinless and boneless
- ½ green bell pepper, chopped
- ½ yellow bell pepper, chopped
- ½ red bell pepper, chopped

Directions:
1. In your Slow cooker, mix tomato sauce with parmesan, onion, garlic, basil, oregano, salt, pepper, chicken, green bell pepper, yellow bell pepper and red bell pepper, toss, cover and cook on Low for 4 hours.
2. Divide between plates and serve for lunch.

Nutrition: calories 221, fat 6, fiber 3, carbs 16, protein 26

Salsa Chicken

Preparation time: 10 minutes
Cooking time: 8 hours
Servings: 2

Ingredients:
- 7 ounces mild salsa
- 1 pound chicken breast, skinless, boneless and cubed
- 1 small yellow onion, chopped
- ½ teaspoon coriander, ground
- ½ teaspoon rosemary, dried
- 1 green bell pepper, chopped
- Cooking spray
- 1 tablespoon cilantro, chopped
- 1 red bell pepper, chopped
- 1 tablespoon chili powder

Directions:
1. Grease the slow cooker with the cooking spray and mix the chicken with the salsa, onion and the other ingredients inside.
2. Put the lid on, cook on Low for 8 hours, divide into bowls and serve for lunch.

Nutrition: calories 240, fat 3, fiber 7, carbs 17, protein 8

Chicken Tacos

Preparation time: 10 minutes
Cooking time: 5 hours
Servings: 16

Ingredients:
- 2 mangos, peeled and chopped
- 2 tomatoes, chopped
- 1 and ½ cups pineapple chunks
- 1 red onion, chopped
- 2 small green bell peppers, chopped
- 1 tablespoon lime juice
- 2 green onions, chopped
- 1 teaspoon sugar
- 4 pounds chicken breast halves, skinless
- Salt and black pepper to the taste
- 32 taco shells, warm
- ¼ cup cilantro, chopped
- ¼ cup brown sugar

Directions:
1. In a bowl, mix mango with pineapple, red onion, tomatoes, bell peppers, green onions and lime juice and toss.
2. Put chicken in your Slow cooker, add salt, pepper and sugar and toss.
3. Add mango mix, cover and cook on Low for 5 hours.
4. Transfer chicken to a cutting board, cool it down, discard bones and shred meat.
5. Divide meat and mango mix between taco shells and serve them for lunch.

Nutrition: calories 246, fat 7, fiber 2, carbs 25, protein 21

Turkey and Mushrooms

Preparation time: 10 minutes
Cooking time: 7 hours and 10 minutes
Servings: 2

Ingredients:
- 1 red onion, sliced
- 2 garlic cloves, minced
- 1 pound turkey breast, skinless, boneless and cubed
- 1 tablespoon olive oil
- 1 teaspoon oregano, dried
- 1 teaspoon basil, dried
- A pinch of red pepper flakes
- 1 cup mushrooms, sliced
- ¼ cup chicken stock
- ½ cup canned tomatoes, chopped
- A pinch of salt and black pepper

Directions:
1. Heat up a pan with the oil over medium-high heat, add the onion , garlic and the meat, brown for 10 minutes and transfer to the slow cooker.
2. Add the oregano, basil and the other ingredients, toss, put the lid on and cook on Low for 7 hours.
3. Divide into bowls and serve for lunch.

Nutrition: calories 240, fat 4, fiber 6, carbs 18, protein 10

Orange Beef Dish

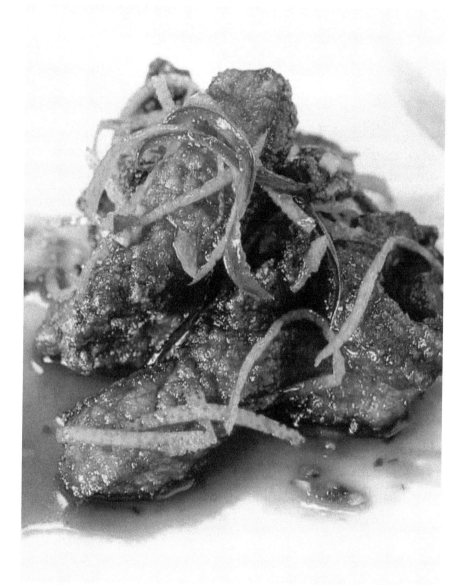

Preparation time: 10 minutes
Cooking time: 5 hours
Servings: 5

Ingredients:

- 1 pound beef sirloin steak, cut into medium strips
- 2 and ½ cups shiitake mushrooms, sliced
- 1 yellow onion, cut into medium wedges
- 3 red hot chilies, dried
- ¼ cup brown sugar
- ¼ cup orange juice
- ¼ cup soy sauce

- 2 tablespoons cider vinegar
- 1 tablespoon cornstarch
- 1 tablespoon ginger, grated
- 1 tablespoon sesame oil
- 1 cup snow peas
- 2 garlic cloves, minced
- 1 tablespoon orange zest, grated

Directions:
1. In your Slow cooker, mix steak strips with mushrooms, onion, chilies, sugar, orange juice, soy sauce, vinegar, cornstarch, ginger, oil, garlic and orange zest, toss, cover and cook on Low for 4 hours and 30 minutes.
2. Add snow peas, cover, cook on Low for 30 minutes more, divide between plates and serve.

Nutrition: calories 310, fat 7, fiber 4, carbs 26, protein 33

Indian Chicken and Tomato Mix

Preparation time: 10 minutes
Cooking time: 6 hours
Servings: 2

Ingredients:
- 1 cup cherry tomatoes, halved
- 1 pound chicken breast, skinless, boneless and cubed
- 1 red onion, sliced
- 1 tablespoons garam masala
- 1 garlic clove, minced
- ½ small yellow onion, chopped
- ½ teaspoon ginger powder
- A pinch of salt and cayenne pepper
- ½ teaspoon sweet paprika
- 2 tablespoons chives, chopped

Directions:
1. In your slow cooker, mix the chicken with the tomatoes, onion and the other ingredients, toss, put the lid on and cook on Low for 6 hours.
2. Divide into bowls and serve right away.

Nutrition: calories 259, fat 3, fiber 7, carbs 17, protein 14

Chicken with Couscous

Preparation time: 10 minutes
Cooking time: 3 hours
Servings: 6

Ingredients:
- 2 sweet potatoes, peeled and cubed
- 1 sweet red peppers, chopped
- 1 and ½ pounds chicken breasts, skinless and boneless
- 13 ounces canned stewed tomatoes
- Salt and black pepper to the taste
- ¼ cup raisins
- ¼ teaspoon cinnamon powder
- ¼ teaspoon cumin, ground

For the couscous:
- 1 cup whole wheat couscous
- 1 cup water
- Salt to the taste

Directions:
1. In your Slow cooker, mix potatoes with red peppers, chicken, tomatoes, salt, pepper, raisins, cinnamon and cumin, toss, cover, cook on Low for 3 hours and shred meat using 2 forks.
2. Meanwhile, heat up a pan with the water over medium-high heat, add salt, bring water to a boil, add couscous, stir, leave aside covered for 10 minutes and fluff with a fork.
3. Divide chicken mix between plates, add couscous on the side and serve.

Nutrition: calories 351, fat 4, fiber 7, carbs 45, protein 30

Turkey and Figs

Preparation time: 10 minutes
Cooking time: 8 hours
Servings: 2

Ingredients:
- 1 pound turkey breast, boneless, skinless and sliced
- ½ cup black figs, halved
- 1 red onion, sliced
- ½ cup tomato sauce
- ½ teaspoon onion powder
- ¼ teaspoon garlic powder
- 1 tablespoon basil, chopped
- ½ teaspoon chili powder
- ¼ cup white wine
- ½ teaspoon thyme, dried
- ¼ teaspoon sage, dried
- ½ teaspoon paprika, dried
- A pinch of salt and black pepper

Directions:
1. In your slow cooker, mix the turkey breast with the figs, onion and the other ingredients, toss, put the lid on and cook on Low for 8 hours.
2. Divide between plates and serve.

Nutrition: calories 220, fat 5, fiber 8, carbs 18, protein 15

Pork Stew

Preparation time: 10 minutes
Cooking time: 5 hours
Servings: 8

Ingredients:
- 2 pork tenderloins, cubed
- Salt and black pepper to the taste
- 2 carrots, sliced
- 1 yellow onion, chopped
- 2 celery ribs, chopped
- 2 tablespoons tomato paste
- 3 cups beef stock
- 1/3 cup plums, dried, pitted and chopped
- 1 rosemary spring
- 1 thyme spring
- 2 bay leaves
- 4 garlic cloves, minced
- 1/3 cup green olives, pitted and sliced
- 1 tablespoon parsley, chopped

Directions:
1. In your Slow cooker, mix pork with salt, pepper, carrots, onion, celery, tomato paste, stock, plums, rosemary, thyme, bay leaves, garlic, olives and parsley, cover and cook on Low for 5 hours.
2. Discard thyme, rosemary and bay leaves, divide stew into bowls and serve for lunch.

Nutrition: calories 200, fat 4, fiber 2, carbs 8, protein 23

Turkey and Walnuts

Preparation time: 10 minutes
Cooking time: 8 hours
Servings: 2

Ingredients:
- 1 pound turkey breast, skinless, boneless and sliced
- ½ cup scallions, chopped
- 2 tablespoons walnuts, chopped
- 1 tablespoon lemon juice
- ¼ cup veggie stock
- ½ teaspoon chili powder
- 1 tablespoon olive oil
- 1 tablespoon rosemary, chopped
- Salt and black pepper to the taste

Directions:
1. In your slow cooker, mix the turkey with the scallions, walnuts and the other ingredients, toss, put the lid on and cook on Low for 8 hours.
2. Divide everything between plates and serve.

Nutrition: calories 264, fat 4, fiber 6, carbs 15, protein 15

Seafood Stew

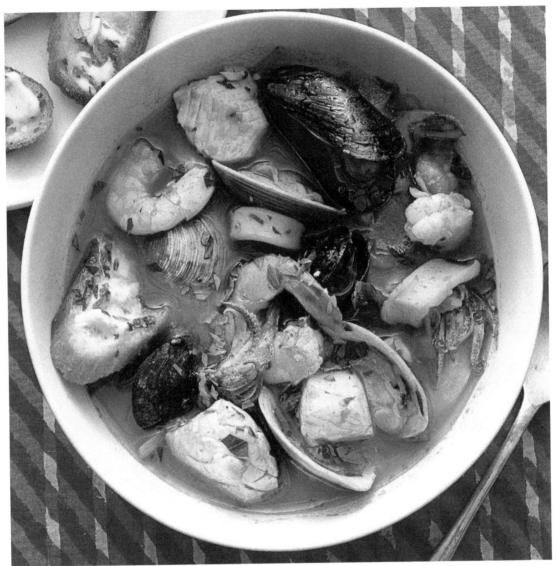

Preparation time: 10 minutes
Cooking time: 4 hours and 30 minutes
Servings: 8

Ingredients:
- 8 ounces clam juice
- 2 yellow onions, chopped
- 28 ounces canned tomatoes, chopped
- 6 ounces tomato paste
- 3 celery ribs, chopped
- ½ cup white wine
- 1 tablespoon red vinegar
- 5 garlic cloves, minced

- 1 tablespoon olive oil
- 1 teaspoon Italian seasoning
- 1 bay leaf
- 1 pound haddock fillets, boneless and cut into medium pieces
- ½ teaspoon sugar
- 1 pound shrimp, peeled and deveined
- 6 ounces crabmeat
- 6 ounces canned clams
- 2 tablespoons parsley, chopped

Directions:

1. In your Slow cooker, mix tomatoes with onions, clam juice, tomato paste, celery, wine, vinegar, garlic, oil, seasoning, sugar and bay leaf, stir, cover and cook on Low for 4 hours.
2. Add shrimp, haddock, crabmeat and clams, cover, cook on Low for 30 minutes more, divide into bowls and serve with parsley sprinkled on top.

Nutrition: calories 205, fat 4, fiber 4, carbs 14, protein 27

Slow Cooked Thyme Chicken

Preparation time: 10 minutes
Cooking time: 7 hours
Servings: 2

Ingredients:
- 1 pound chicken legs
- 1 tablespoon thyme, chopped
- 2 garlic cloves, minced
- ½ cup chicken stock
- 1 carrot, chopped
- ½ yellow onion, chopped
- A pinch of salt and white pepper
- Juice of ½ lemon

Directions:
1. In your slow cooker, mix the chicken legs with the thyme, garlic and the other ingredients, toss, put the lid on and cook on Low for 7 hours.
2. Divide between plates and serve.

Nutrition: calories 320, fat 4, fiber 7, carbs 16, protein 6

Conclusion

Did you enjoy trying these new and also delightful meals? sadly we have actually come to the end of this slow-moving cooker cookbook, I absolutely want it has really been to your liking. to boost your health as well as wellness we would enjoy to advise you to include exercise as well as also a dynamic means of living together with comply with these excellent recipes, so as to highlight the improvements. we will definitely be back quickly with various other considerably fascinating vegan recipes, a large hug, see you soon.

CPSIA information can be obtained
at www.ICGtesting.com
Printed in the USA
LVHW060005260521
688447LV00017B/928